The secret to perfect health

Tony Davis,P.H.T.
(Perfect Health Teacher)
HOW TO ENJOY PERFECT HEALTH FOREVER

To order additional copies of this breakthrough book, please go to www.amazon.com They are $10 each.

GOT PROOF?
Everything I wrote in this book is true and I'm gonna prove it to you!
Everything I wrote in this unique unprecedented book is backed up by facts and by scientific proof!

NOTE:All the sayings in my book were invented by me unless otherwise specified. Also,certain names have been changed to protect people's privacy.

For updates of this book visit: **www.happyforever.us**
TABLE OF CONTENTS

DEDICATION

I dedicate this book to mankind:

God's ultimate creation of all time!

Here are 10 reasons why I love mankind more than anybody in the world:

1-Humans are a perfect creation in every way imaginable

2-Humans are the most amazing creation that God ever created

3-Humans are a unique,superb,breakthrough creation

4-Humans are the most beautiful creation on Earth and probably in the entire universe

5-Humans are the most intelligent creation on planet Earth and the intelligence they possess is infinite

6-Women are the most precious creation because they continue life-No pregnancy=no more humanity

7-Women are the most magical creation because they can make a man happy in at least 69 different ways

8-Humans are able to experience the most powerful pleasure in the universe: have sex or make love

9-Humans are able to create whatever they imagine

10-Humans are divine beings with unlimited potential

PREFACE

We live in a world where most people are unhappy. You <u>can</u> be happy forever,you just need to know how. You need to know a lot of secrets and I'll tell you all the secrets possible to help you enjoy permanent happiness. After reading my book you can be happy forever. I can tell you from the bottom of my golden heart that my book is one of the best books you will ever read or even the best. It contains information that will blow your mind. Unique and exciting new information that will change your life forever. Information that will make you happier than ever. I will tell you exactly what you need to do to,step by step,to be happy forever. I'll also tell you what is keeping you from enjoying everlasting happiness.

A lot of the information contained in this book is not found in any other book and I predict that this book will change the future of humanity for better,for good and forever. Do you know why 99% of the people on this planet are not happy forever? Because they don't believe they can or they don't know how or both.

DISCLAIMER

Everything I wrote in this book is strictly my opinion. However, everything I wrote in this book I based it on facts and hard scientific evidence. The information in this book is for educational purposes only. It does not constitute medical advice and should not be construed as such. I cannot guarantee the safety and effectiveness of any treatment, remedy or advice mentioned. Some of the tips may not be effective for everyone. A good medical doctor is the best judge of what medical treatment may be needed for certain conditions and diseases. I strongly recommend that in all cases you contact your personal medical doctor or health care provider before changing your diet or discontinuing any medication you are taking or before treating yourself in any way. I am not making an attempt to prescribe any medical treatment. I am not responsible in any way, shape or form for any bad consequences you might experience from taking my advice. My book is not intended to treat, prevent or cure any disease. The information provided in this book is designed to provide helpful information on the subjects discussed. This book is not meant to be used, nor should it be used, to diagnose or treat any medical condition. For diagnosis or treatment of any medical problem, consult your own physician. The publisher and author are not responsible for any specific health or allergy needs that may require medical supervision and are not liable for any damages or negative consequences from any treatment, action, application or preparation to any person reading or following the information in this book. References are provided for informational purposes only and do not constitute endorsement of any websites or other sources.

CHAPTER ONE:
HOW TO ENJOY PERFECT HEALTH

When it comes to eliminating all your health problems that are bothering you now,you have choices but before I tell you about your choices,there is a major serious health problem which makes a lot of people suffer for a long period of time and it's called pain. If you are in pain,no matter how long you've been in pain and you want pain relief in a few seconds or a few minutes I got some real natural no drugs pain relief good news for you:

Lifewave products.

Please visit:www.lifewave.com for more info.

Go there and see how you can finally live pain free.

WARNING: If you are taking pain killers aka pain drugs for your pain you are making a deadly mistake.

"Pain killers are killers"

Fact:

"Pain killers kill your pain but they also kill you"

Painkillers are killing around 15,000 people per year.

When it comes to eliminating all your health problems,you have 3 options:

OPTION#1:I will teach you for free how

OPTION#2:See a natural doctor

OPTION#3:You do it yourself

OPTION#1:I will teach you for free how

I am a perfect health teacher so you can email me and I will tell you step by step what you need to do to eliminate forever any health problem or problems that are bothering you. I can help you even if you are broke because my price is very good for your health:

I'm in charge so no charge! Your health is more important to me. Making you healthy makes me happy.

What price? I don't need the money. I'm rich! I will also give you my cell number when you email me and I will help you for free and for ever!Also,I will do the same for all the people you love and care about!And I am very happy to do it with all my golden heart! I'm enjoying perfect health every day and now it's time for you to enjoy it,too! And of course,it's up to you.

OPTION#2:See a natural doctor

You have many choices when it comes to seeing a natural doctor and I'll give the 10 best choices I found so far:

CHOICE#1:Fasting

CHOICE#2:See a natural doctor like a:

a)Naturopath

b)Homeopath

c)Acupuncturist

d)Herbalist

e)Iridologist

f)Hypnotist

CHOICE#3:Dermatron Machine

CHOICE#4:Bio-resonance

CHOICE#5:Oxygen Therapy

CHOICE#6:Ozone Therapy

CHOICE#7:Stem Cell Therapy

CHOICE#8:Pranic Healing

CHOICE#9:Theta Healing

CHOICE#10:The pH of the body

CHOICE#1:FASTING

"The fastest way to perfect health is fasting"

What is fasting?

Fasting is a period of abstinence from all food. When you fast you don't eat any food,you only drink water or juices or both.

During the absence of food the body will systematically cleanse itself of everything except vital tissue. Although protein is being used by the body during the fast,a person fasting even for 30 days on water only will not suffer a deficiency of protein,vitamins,minerals or fatty acids. When fasting,a person experiences recovery at a rate that is much faster than normal.

He or she is ridding his or her body of toxins and excesses,allowing the body to use its own wisdom to healthfully reorganize itself from the atomic level. While the toxic load is reduced, the functioning of every cell is improved. Virtually everyone who fasts discovers the same thing,that when they fast they actually have no hunger and more energy than they usually have. It is very exciting to find out that if we let our bodies do their job,most or all of our health problems will disappear.

The body is healing itself 24/7:when you are up and when you sleep. Fasting is the simplest,easiest and most effective way to find out that we do have the power and freedom to heal our bodies and take control of our health. Fasting has been practiced for at least 10,000 years and it is the fastest and cheapest way to perfect health.

What fasting could do for you:

1-Mental clarity is improved and brain fog is gone

2-Rapid and safe weight loss is achieved without flabbiness and the weight stays off

3-The nervous system is balanced

4-Energy level and sensory perception is increased The longer the fast,the bigger increase in energy and vitality

5-Organs are revitalized and rejuvenated

6-Cellular biochemistry is harmonized

7-The skin becomes young looking,soft and clear

8-Breathing becomes fuller,freer and deeper
9-The digestive system is rejuvenated and becomes more effective and the natural bowel movement is normalized after fasting
10-As soon as the body realizes that it's fasting it will begin to eliminate those things that cause disease,such as fat cells,arterial cholesterol plaques,mucus,tumors,stored up worries and emotions,etc.

If you decide to fast,there are many fasting clinics out there but here is one I recommend because it is the cheapest and the best in the world and you can fast from home,no matter what country you live in:
www.fasting.com

WARNING:NEVER ever do any kind of fasting unless supervised by a fasting professional practitioner.

CHOICE#2:SEE A NATURAL PRACTITIONER LIKE A:

a)Naturopath
b)Homeopath
c)Acupuncturist
d)Herbalist
e)Iridologist
f)Hypnotist

a)A NATUROPATH

Naturopathic medicine treats all forms of health concerns:from pediatric to geriatric,from irritating systems to chronic illness and from the physical to the psychological. It is the approach,philosophy and training of the naturopathic doctors that makes them better than other forms of natural treatment. Who should see a naturopathic doctor? People that are looking for disease prevention and for natural ways to keep the body healthy

Individuals that have already realized that health doesn't just happen by chance and it is a life-long process that involves a clear understanding of the things that make you sick and how to avoid them on a daily basis. People that have an array of symptoms that they have been unable to address on their own or
with the help of their own incapable medical doctors. With naturopathic medicine's broad understanding of health and the relationship between health,life and the environment, naturopathic doctors are often able to offer patients hope and provide natural,safe and effective ways to restore perfect health.People that have been diagnosed with an illness and are looking for natural alternative treatments. Naturopathic medicine is very effective in improving the quality of life for those with serious and life threatening diseases It is used extensively and effectively for people that are looking to combine common sense and naturopathic treatments with the goal of eliminating the devastating side effects of drugs,vaccines or surgery which are all toxic and many deadly. The naturopathic philosophy is to stimulate the innate healing power of the body and to treat the actual cause of disease and not to treat the symptoms like medical doctors do. By finding out the real cause of disease and through the adequate use of natural therapies many people eliminated their health problems meaning they got cured.
For more information visit:
www.naturopathy.com
b)A HOMEOPATH
Homeopathic doctors work in the same way as any other natural doctors do. Careful examination and investigation are very important in establishing the diagnosis.

Besides asking about your symptoms,a homeopathic doctor will also be interested in you as an individual and the unique way in which your symptoms affect your health. He or she will ask you questions about your lifestyle, your eating habits,your drinking habits,your smoking habits,your stress level,your temperament,your personality, your family and friends that could affect your health,your sleeping habits and your medical history which will help the doctor to form a complete picture of you. This picture will be matched to the symptoms of your illness in order to prescribe a particular type and strength of homeopathic remedy that is unique to you.After the diagnosis is made,your homeopathic doctor will give you a natural prescription. Homeopathy is usually taken in tablets or capsules but is also available in liquid and powder form. You may be prescribed a homeopathic gel or cream for topical use,also. All homeopathic remedies are natural and they have no side effects.They are actually herbs and plants and they can cure you. For more information visit: www.homeopathy.com

c)AN ACUPUNCTURIST

Acupuncture is a method of helping the body to promote natural healing and to unblock the energy flow in the body. This is done by inserting needles at very precise acupuncture points. A good acupuncturist will give you unique powerful herbs too in addition to the needles. What? You got a question? Ask way! What the hell is acupuncture? Answer:The classical Chinese explanation is that channels of energy run in regular patterns through the body and over its surface. These energy channels, called meridians are like rivers flowing through the body to irrigate and nourish the tissues.

An obstacle in the movement of these energy rivers is like a dam that backs up in others.

The meridians can be influenced by needling the acupuncture points. The acupuncture needles unblock the obstacles at the dams and reestablish the regular flow through the meridians. Acupuncture treatments help the body's internal organs to correct imbalances in their digestion,absorption and energy production activities and in the circulation of their energy through the meridians. The modern scientific explanation is that needling the acupuncture points stimulates the nervous system to release chemicals in the muscles,spinal cord and brain. These chemicals will either change the experience of pain or they will trigger the release of other chemicals and hormones which influence the body's own internal regulating system. The improved energy and biochemical balance produced by acupuncture results in the body's natural healing abilities to be activated faster and in promoting physical and emotional well-being. Acupuncture is a system which can influence three areas of healthcare:

Area#1:Promotion of health and well-being
Area#2:Prevention of disease
Area#3:Healing many medical conditions

Many times acupuncture is used on patients that are in pain. Acupuncture can be effective as the only treatment used or as the support to other natural treatments. Acupuncture is specifically useful in solving physical problems related to tension,stress and emotional conditions. In the past 5,000 years,more people have been successfully treated with acupuncture than with all other treatments combined.

Acupuncture is successfully used all over the world and it is now being used more and more in America by patients and natural doctors.

Acupuncture treatments can be given at the same time other natural treatments are being used. Make sure that you let your acupuncturist know about any other natural treatments you are getting so you can get the most benefit from all your treatments. Some acupuncturists will also give you strong herbs from Asia in addition to the needles to speed up your healing process.

For more information visit:

www.acupuncture.com

d)AN HERBALIST

Herbal medicine is the traditional Chinese and Korean use of plant remedies in the treatment of disease. It is the oldest and most natural form of medicine known to man. Our ancestors used the most effective local plants to heal their ailments. Today we combine that knowledge with cutting edge research,analytical chemistry and modern medical science. Many scientific clinical trials of herbal medicines are being conducted all over the world with results that are surprising the uneducated medical doctors who do not know anything about herbal medicines. Herbal medicine is a very popular practiced form of medicine in the world with over 69% of the world's population relying on the proven and effective use of herbs for healing virtually any disease. Herbalists use pure whole plant herbal remedies not plant based concentrated or standardized extracts. Plants contain thousands of constituents,active constituents being balanced within the plant by many other substances which make them more powerful.

Herbalists have time to really listen and discuss your problems and they are not limited to 5 minutes as some over-worked medical doctors are. Herbalists take a holistic view of illness.

The underlying imbalance in the body as a whole is sought and it is this that is treated not just the symptoms alone. They are gentle but very effective and have no side effects unlike prescribed drugs. They may take longer to act as they work to restore the balance of the body enabling it to heal itself from within. The herbal prescriptions are unique for each person. It is the person that is treated not the disease. So although certain herbs have an affinity for particular organs or systems of the body,it is highly unlikely that any two people will ever receive the same prescription or dosage. Herbal Medicine can also be used to help in preventing illness by strengthening and balancing the body and mind so that health is naturally maintained. According to my research one of the best herbs in the world can be found here: www.herbdoc.com

e)AN IRIDOLOGIST

I am gonna ask you an easy question: How many eyes do you have? I'll make this easier for you: How much is one plus one? That's how many eyes you have! Two! Now the hard question: How many functions do the eyes have? If you think the eyes have only one function, think again:

Two eyes=Two functions

Coin-cidence?

Let's flip a coin and find out! Say what? Let's not? OK! Yes,my esteemed friends,colleagues and comrades:

The eyes have 2 functions:

1-The first one is for seeing

2-The second one is for storage

1-Seeing

You use your eyes every day to see everything around you including good stuff like hot women!
And even cold women!

2-Storage

Everything that is going on in your body and in your brain is stored in your eyes. When I say everything,I am talking about your health,of course. If you're healthy,an iridologist will see that in your eyes. If you're sick,the iridologist will see that too.Iridology is the science of analyzing the color and structure of the eye to determine tissue integrity throughout the body to gain valuable health information about your body and your mind. If you have a medical mystery,a mysterious health problem or a mysterious disease,then I suggest you see an iridologist because they will look into your eyes and tell you exactly what's wrong with you. I saw an iridologist myself and I was very impressed with the results. Even if you are healthy or think that you're healthy,you should see an iridologist. Iridology is one form of analysis that is non-invasive to the body requiring no cutting,no x-raying and no using of any other invasive technique which is dangerous or deadly to your precious health. By looking into our eyes,an iridologist can reveal our inherited health disposition,our tendency towards health problems,our current health conditions and they also give advance warning of what may occur in the future.

No other natural doctor can do that!
Today when the health of humanity is worse than ever,early detection of health issues and immediate correction is vitally important. Iridology is a tool for evaluating current conditions and for preventive healthcare.

A practitioner skilled in iris analysis uses either a hand held light source and a small magnifying lens or for more extensive analysis a special camera is used for taking prints,slides or digital pictures allowing the practitioner the ability to study the iris at length before completing the analysis.

(The iris is the big circle part of your eye).

Iridology is at least 5,000 years old and it is used worldwide with amazingly accurate results.

After you see an iridologist,you will be given natural treatment to heal you. If you decide to see an iridologist when can look for one in your area and if you live in California,contact me and I'll give you the name and number of the best iridologist I found so far:

My own personal iridologist!

PS:When I went to see an iridologist in my country Romania,my health was the worst ever. I was severely depressed,I was in pain,I was pissed because I didn't know what was wrong with me after seeing a lot of medical doctors. That is a mistake I will never make!

My Romanian iridologist looked into my eyes for only one minute or less and what he told me changed my life forever. First of all he told me that there is nothing wrong with my body or my brain. Second he told me that he has never seen such a brilliant brain like mine. He said that my brain is similar to Albert Einstein's brain. He told me that I have the brain of a genius! Third of all,he gave me an example about my brain being different than most people's brains. Then he gave me a hypothetical example so I can get a clearer picture about my genius brain.

He said that my brain speed is 1,300 km per hour and normal people's brain speed is 900 km per hour.

So my brain thinks faster by 400 km per hour than most people's brains. That was one of the best news I have ever received in my entire life!

Finally he prescribed me some herbs and plants and my depression and my pain were history after 6 months.

Later on I found out that my Romanian iridologist was the best in Romania and one of the best in Europe!

If you want to pay him a visit,you only have to pay him $20 for a consultation!

However,if you live in another country,the plane ticket ain't gonna be that cheap!Anyway,what's more important: Your money or your health?

However,you can see an iridologist that is close to where you live and it won't break your bank!

For more info you can also check out: www.iridology.com

f)A HYPNOTIST

What can a hypnotist do for you? I could answer that question by writing a very long list but that would be boring to read! Because of that I will supply you with a short list of the most common things that hypnosis is used to treat:phobias like spiders,snakes,height, public speaking,etc. Hypnosis also treats bad habits,smoking cessation,anxiety,sports performance, sexual issues,pain and chronic pain,panic,weight loss,gain and maintenance,relationship problems, personal goal achievement,birthing problems, pre and post operative relaxation problems,how to do past life regression and much more. Hypnosis is often used when all regular treatments have failed. A lot of problems seems to stem from unconscious limiting beliefs. These limiting beliefs can sometimes prevent you from spelling well,reading well,performing well in the you suck,oops,in the sack and so on. Since they are unconscious limiting beliefs you don't know that you have them so how can you know if hypnosis could be helpful to you?

You don't,but you can call up a hypnotist and ask for their opinion. You can also visit:www.hypnosis.edu

CHOICE#3: THE DERMATRON MACHINE

Imagine if you could go to your natural doctor,sit for an hour in a comfortable chair where you are hooked up to some highly sophisticated electronic equipment which is painless and then receive a detailed assessment of your health status. Sounds too good to be true? It sound that way but it is 100% true. Maybe,thousands of progressive practitioners around the world are already providing this service. Not only can these practitioners provide an in-depth health assessment but they can also treat many problems right on the spot with electrical impulses and can prescribe safe and very specific natural remedies for conditions which take longer to cure.

The Dermatron machine or the "energy machine" is used not only to establish specific diagnoses but also to determine food allergies and the presence of toxins in the body. This miraculous machine is also used to determine the exact remedies required to correct any health problems. A significant number of the more than 3000 acupoints corresponding to specific parts of the internal organs are being tested during a consultation. During testing the patient holds an electrode in their hand but here the practitioner makes the primary diagnosis by pressing a pointed probe against many different acupoints representing internal organs and their specific parts.

Some of the more sophisticated machines are also capable of assessing heart and brain functions and can provide specific information about the state of individual parts of the endocrine,digestive and immune system.

The Dermatron machine is a breakthrough machine and can quickly diagnose your health problem within minutes,not hours like ordinary medical doctors who take so many tests,it takes days to get those results.

The energy machine can give you your results in just a few minutes and then the Dermatron Machine practitioner can give you the adequate natural treatment and you can start your road to perfect health!

Here's a website that has all the practitioners from all over the world:

http://reenie.org/site/electro/practitioners.html

CHOICE#4:BIO-RESONANCE

Bio-resonance has been in mainstream medical use for more than two decades in many countries around the world. The diagnosing possibilities of the technology are such that it is possible not only to define the character of disease but to optimize its treatment.

The list of diseases being treated successfully is huge. All matter has a resonant frequency and every cell in the body resonates at a particular frequency. This takes the form of an electromagnetic field. Groups of cells in an organ or system have multiple frequency patterns which are unique. The whole body has a complex frequency make-up,which can be changed or distorted by disease.

Because the cells are controlled by electromagnetic fields,it is then possible to introduce healthy frequencies to re-balance the whole body and provide an environment in which the body can cure itself. Your body resonates at certain 'normal' electromagnetic frequencies.

Toxic substances like chemicals,heavy metals and

poisons (like prescribed drugs and vaccines),alter the body's 'normal' vibration or frequency pattern.

The body starts to adapt to the new frequency pattern and that is why we get addictions or chronic illness or develop mental or physical conditions through exposure to adverse energies like power cables, mobile phones and computers.

This unhealthy frequency becomes 'you' while the toxin remains in the body. These toxic frequencies are removed with the Bio-resonance Technology. Modifying and correcting subtle energy patterns so the body is allowed to return back to its 'normal' healthy status. This process has already helped many people become addiction free,allergy free,infection free,pain free and disease free. Bio-resonance treatment helps the body's own regulation and detoxification system, boosts the body's natural immune system which is the single most important part of any healing method.

The Bio-resonance system used by the clinics around the world is one of the most advanced,if not the most advanced in the global marketplace and has within it access to more than 300,000 different remedies.

Bio-resonance is used as a therapeutic measure or in other words it is an influence of small electromagnetic fluctuations which are generated by a device and it can be compared to the way modern cars are now diagnosed. It is simply being connected to a device that checks your system for imbalances and then corrects those imbalances. It can only produce beneficial results with zero side effects. Bio-resonance is a treatment which quite simply releases those areas within our body that are blocking the natural energy flow of the body.

Bio-resonance allows reduction or complete removal of any medication (poison) you might be taking and restores the affected balance of the body.

Bio-resonance is often used as an alternative way when it is found impossible to solve your health problems with the help of conventional therapy which is usually a toxic treatment:medication or surgery which is ineffective and very dangerous to your health or deadly.

Bio-resonance testing represents an important diagnostic breakthrough of modern medicine and perhaps the most significant in the history of medical diagnosis. It is not a method yet accepted into mainstream medical practice because your own doctor doesn't want you to get well.

He wants you to be sick so you can keep seeing him or your medical doctor will be out of business in no time if you and all his patients were in perfect health.

There is an ill saying:

"A pill for every ill"

That's what your medical doctor is doing to you:giving you a pill for every ill or he is treating your symptoms. Your medical doctor doesn't heal you and he never will because pills,vaccines and surgery are a barbaric treatment against humanity but it sure makes a lot people a lot of money. Billions of dollars in profit to be exact.

The money is in treating people not healing them

That's why they never found a cure for any disease and they never will because only your own body can cure yourself but keep lying to us on TV that a cure is around the corner. Around the corner in hell,I say!

However, Bio-resonance is popular among natural and alternative medical practitioners worldwide. In my opinion it is set to rise in popularity as one of the most useful of all diagnostic techniques of all time.

Here are the major advantages of Bio-resonance testing:
a)Non-invasive,therefore no side effects
b)Ability to pinpoint exact information concerning the state of internal organs and harmful factors lodged in them,including many organs and tissues normally inaccessible to diagnostic investigation except under conditions of autopsy like postmortem examination
c)The capability to investigate the levels of stress and toxicity and/or strain due to other deadly factors in the many body compartments(the organs and the tissues). The kind of information gathered is not a disease label nor the ruling out of a disease label. It is therefore an accurate diagnostic tool for those interested in assessing organ health,toxicity level,stress levels and eventually perfect health!

On the following website you will find a list of bio-resonance practitioners from around the world: http://www.informationenergymedicine-association.com/laeser-bioresonance-practitioners

CHOICE#5: OXYGEN THERAPY

Oxygen therapy is a treatment that provides you with extra oxygen,a gas that is vital for your body to be healthy. Normally, your lungs absorb oxygen from the air. As you already know,the air we breathe is not clean. However, that depends in what part of the world you live. There are few cities or villages in the world where people breathe clean air. Still,that's not enough. Many diseases can prevent you from getting enough oxygen.

Oxygen therapy helps you eliminate some of your health problems or all of them. Oxygen therapy can be done in a hospital or at home. If you need oxygen therapy for a chronic disease or condition, you should receive home oxygen therapy. Your natural doctor will decide if you need oxygen therapy based on the results of some tests,such as an arterial blood gas test and a pulse oximetry test. These tests measure how much oxygen is in your blood. A low oxygen level is a sign that you need oxygen therapy. Oxygen is considered a medicine,so your doctor must prescribe it.

Oxygen therapy helps many people function better and be more active. It also may help decrease shortness of breath and fatigue. It can also improve sleep in some people who have sleep-related breathing disorders and increase the lifespan of some people who have COPD. If you don't know what COPD means,then you don't need to worry about it because you don't have it!

Although you may need oxygen therapy long term, it doesn't have to limit your daily routine. Portable oxygen units can make it easier for you to move around and do many daily activities. Talk with your natural doctor if you have questions about the safety of certain activities while you are getting oxygen therapy. A home equipment provider will work with you to make sure you have the supplies and equipment you need. Trained professionals will also show you how to use the equipment correctly and safely. Oxygen therapy generally is safe but it can pose a fire hazard. In order to use your oxygen safely,follow the instructions you receive from your home equipment provider. There are many oxygen therapy practitioners but the one I recommend is: www.whitakerwellness.com

CHOICE#6: OZONE THERAPY

Ozone Therapy is a medical therapy that has been used worldwide for over 75 years with tremendous success. In some clinics around the world ,ozone is the first agent given to each and every patient that enters the clinic regardless of their illnesses. Ozone addresses the key issues in almost all diseases.

Ozone therapy has proven beneficial effects such as: increasing oxygen delivery to cells, tissues, and organs increasing blood circulation throughout the body, detoxification, boosting of the immune system,sterilizing and healing external wounds (many of which would otherwise heal much slower) gangrene and much more.

For more information you can visit: http://www.ozoneuniversity.com

CHOICE#7-STEM CELL THERAPY

The discovery of adult stem cell therapy has been a medical breakthrough because how effective this method is in curing a number of diseases. Adult stem cells come from a number of biological sources such as:blood,umbilical cords,bone marrow, muscle,placenta,fat,breast milk,dental pulp,etc.

It has been discovered that these adult stem cells act as the body's natural healing cells which is why they are used to heal a number of diseases that modern medical medicine has been unable to cure. The number one advantage about using adult stem cells is that there are virtually no side effects. It has been used for over 50 years in the treatment of cancer and research has shown that it has also been effective in the treatment of over 500 diseases. Stem cells can divide indefinitely as long as required to repair and replenish other cells. Once a stem cell has divided,it may either remain the same or it can the become another type of cell. Stem cells are effective in curing disease because of their unique ability to support to other cells in the body. They also work in our body's tissues to repair any cells that need it.

Besides curing disease,stem cell treatments have been effective in pain management as well as prevention. When it comes to the safety of a stem cell transplant,thy shalt not worry:it is completely safe! Here is a fact for you so you can put your worries to rest and be more confident of stem cell treatment procedures:

None of the stem cell treatments has ever resulted in a negative outcome. Stem cell therapy practices have been carefully designed in order to avoid any complications.

For more information you can visit: www.stemcelltreatmentinstitute.com

CHOICE#8: PRANIC HEALING

Pranic Healing is a very evolved and tested system of energy natural medicine developed by Grand master Chow Lok Zeng that utilizes prana to balance,harmonize and transform the body's energy processes.

Prana is a Sanskrit word that means life-force. This invisible bio-energy or vital energy keeps the body alive and maintains a state of good health. In acupuncture,the Chinese refer to this subtle energy as "Chi"

Pranic Healing is a simple but powerful and effective system energy healing that uses only the hands of the practitioner. (The hands never touch the body).

It is based on the basic principle that the body is a self-repairing living entity that possesses the ability to heal itself and that the healing process is speeded up by increasing this life force that is readily available from the sun,air and ground to correct physical and emotional imbalances. Life Energy or prana is all around us. It is pervasive and we are actually in an ocean of Life Energy. Based on this fact,a healer can draw in Pranic Energy or Life Energy from the surroundings and heal people.

Physical contact is not required because the practitioner is working on the bioplasmic or energy body and not directly on the physical body. This energy body or aura is the mold or blueprint that surrounds and interpenetrates the physical body. It is the energy body that absorbs life energy and distributes it throughout the physical body. The reason Pranic Healing works on the energy body first is because all the physical energy blocks or imbalances first appear as energetic disruptions in the aura before materializing as health problems in the physical body. This pervasive energy that surrounds, interpenetrates and sustains the physical body, also affects our emotions,our ability to handle our jobs,our stress,our relationships,our finances,our health and our happiness. In ancient times, Pranic Healing could only be practiced by an elite few.

Today many effective healing systems were developed,which ordinary people could learn in a short period of time. Anybody can practice pranic healing.

The knowledge of being able to deal with simple ailments is quite empowering. You can be healed or heal other people or both. The courses offered are designed to give a person a well-rounded education in Energy Healing and other Esoteric Sciences. These courses are offered across the United States and all over the world. I welcome you to the Exciting World of Energy and the Pranic Healing System!

PS:If you live in Southern California you can get pranic healing treatments for free here: http://pranichealingusa.com/wordpress or you can search the internet for a location near you where they have free pranic healing sessions.

Good lick,Good suck and Good luck!

CHOICE#9: THETA HEALING

Bringing together the science of Quantum Physics and Metaphysics,Theta Healing can easily and quickly help you solve your health problems. It is a completely new way of healing the body for most people in the world. This healing process will change the way you think and feel about any health challenges forever.

Theta Healing is a powerful,accurate tool for deep and everlasting change in shifting and healing your life on all levels and liberating you from stubborn beliefs,negative beliefs,unrealistic beliefs,destructive patterns of thinking or any kind of pessimistic thinking which can hurt your health. It is unbelievably fast and has already helped thousands of people worldwide. Theta Healing provides a path to effortless change. It is an Energy Healing technique where the healer uses "theta" brain waves to connect to the "Source"(God) and to channel healing energy. It can be used to eliminate beliefs that are keeping you clinging to unwanted habits and hobbies. An old stubborn belief such as "I am not good enough" can be traced quickly to its origins and then transformed into a positive life affirming statement.

Physical illnesses can be cured instantly.
It has been widely used with huge success in all matters of Body,Mind,Spirit and Disease.

Our thoughts (both conscious and unconscious) is the first thing that create our lives. Theta Healing can help you make major changes in your life by releasing negative thoughts that have been in your mind for years,decades or even your entire life. Core beliefs hidden in the subconscious shape your physical,mental and emotional reality without you even knowing it. These beliefs can add positive or negative energy to your life.

The negative energy will affect or destroy your health. Theta Healing can quickly and accurately pinpoint your roadblocks and lift them,allowing you to move easily and confidently towards your goal which is perfect health obviously.

What are subconscious beliefs you asked?

About 90% of how we think is in our subconscious. It is taught to us by our families,our culture,our education and our religions. We learn it early in life before we become capable of conscious thought and reasoning. Theta healing is a process of accessing the Theta brainwave in order to connect with the creative force(the universe) and communicate with the cells in your body to create healing. Healing can be on the emotional level by changing certain core belief programs which are affecting your life or your health or both or healing may be mostly physical by communicating directly with the cells of your body. The Theta Brainwaves are generated when we are asleep,dreaming or under deep hypnosis. It is this frequency that cells use to talk to other cells in the body and this allows us to communicate with our body without interference. It is this interference that causes 'dis-ease' in the body. We have the inherent right to happiness and perfect health. This process allows us to work with the co-creative part of God that is within all of us to create happiness in our lives and ultimately perfect health.

For more information visit:

www.thetahealing.com

CHOICE#10: THE PH OF THE BODY

You want perfect health,right? What are the initials of Perfect Health? P and H,right? Or PH! So far,so good! Coincidentally pH which stands for Potential of Hydrogen and also has the same initials:PH.

Did you know that the pH of your body needs to be 7 if you want to achieve perfect health? What is pH?

pH is an acronym for "potential of Hydrogen" or the acid to alkaline ratio existing in all matter and our 7.365 body pH measurement is the benchmark for measuring our health. Many items have a pH measurement. Here are a few:batteries,swimming pool water and people. The pH scale or chart is typically color coded and ranges from 0 to 14.Anything that tests below 7 is acidic and anything above 7 is alkaline. A healthy person's blood should be a 7 pH. If we move that measurement 2 points either way it can be dangerous or fatal. Our body protects us from that if we start to become too acidic by stealing high pH minerals(from our bones)to neutralize the acidity.

Sometimes it does so much that symptoms, chronic symptoms or disease will follow. A healthy person has a pH that ranges from 6.0 to 7.5 and a sick person has a pH that is below 6.The lower your pH is the sicker you are. The fluids in the cells of most people's bodies are overly acidic. This can cause a lot of serious health problems. It prevents your body from neutralizing toxins and leaves you more susceptible to the cell-damaging free radical oxidation that leads to cancer and other diseases. People with more acidic blood were more likely to be ill.

A pH range of 7.4 to 7.5 to be associated with good health. When foods are metabolized,acids are produced which are neutralized by the alkaline salts (carbonates) of calcium, magnesium, potassium and sodium.

Foods containing chlorine,phosphorous,sulfur and nitrogen, animal products and refined carbohydrates tend to be acid forming. How do you know what your pH is?

You need to test your body pH by testing your urine or saliva. Most likely your pH is below 6 which is unhealthy and you will need specific products to raise your body's pH and make your body alkaline. Email me and I'll tell you exactly which products I'm taking to keep my body alkaline aka healthy. You also have another choice to make your body alkaline:eat foods that are alkaline and drink beverages that are alkaline. Or add them to your daily diet. According to one doctor there is only one disease out there and it's called acidosis. Acidosis is caused by too much acid in the body or too many toxins.

The toxins or the garbage inside our body is not something solid,it is something liquid and the body stores it as acid. The more acid you have in your body the more health problems you are gonna have and if you have a lot of acid in your body then you will get a disease which is created by your own body so the body can eliminate the extra toxins and be clean and healthy again. When it comes to health and disease there is a lot of information out there that is so confusing but fortunately I will make very simple for you because it really is simple to be healthy and stay healthy.

A sick body is an acidic body and a healthy body is an alkaline body

An acidic body has too much acid or toxins. An alkaline body has no toxins and therefore is a healthy body. Unfortunately almost all of us have acidic bodies. How do you know if your body is acidic? If you have just one health problem then your body is acidic or it is deficient in vitamins,minerals,micro-nutrients,etc or both.

Your body is perfect and you should have perfect health It's your birth right. Acidosis is considered by many researchers to be the basic foundation of all diseases. It's a real silent killer. Do you know why heart disease is the number one killer in the world? Because our bodies

are acidic and the acid is making holes in your blood vessels inside your heart. The simple process of alkalizing our body and the important role a properly alkalized body plays in restoring and maintaining our overall health,is paramount in any serious pursuit of wellness. That's because our glands and organs function properly in exact proportion to the amount of alkaline and acid levels in our system. It is estimated that 70 to 80% of what goes into our body is acid-forming and this has a devastating impact on the body's pH. The result of this is decay and putrefaction in the colon,which causes the formation of dangerous acids that affect cells,organs,glands and body functions. As we age,because the entire metabolic process becomes progressively more acid,organ tissues begin to show the signs of stress and damage,
and "dis-ease" is being born. Virtually everybody believes that the older we get,the sicker we get. Not true. The real reason most people get sicker as they get older is because the older they get the more acidic their body becomes. Fact:
Every sick person is over-acidic
If you keep your body alkaline you can enjoy perfect health for the rest of your life and you will also live a long healthy life. Total healing of a chronic illness only takes place when and if the blood is restored to a normal,slightly alkaline pH. The heart is one of the most alkaline-dependent organs in the body. Now you know why heart disease is the number one killer in the world.
Correct heartbeat is altered by acid wastes.
These wastes rob the blood of proper oxygenation,then degeneration of the heart follows and
in many cases instant death or heart attacks.

OPTION#3:In order to eliminate any health problem that you have yourself,you have to do the following 3 things:

1-ELIMINATE ALL THE STRESS FROM YOUR LIFE OR REDUCE IT

2-ELIMINATE THE DEAD FOODS AND BEVERAGES FROM YOUR DIET or MINIMIZE THEM

3-CORRECT THE DEFICIENCIES IN YOUR BODY BY GIVING YOUR BODY WHAT IT NEEDS

1-ELIMINATE THE STRESS FROM YOUR LIFE

The first step you have to take towards perfect health is to eliminate all the stress from your life. Stress is caused by many things like:

a)Money problems

b)Relationship problems

c)The losers in your life

d)Worrying,complaining,fighting,shouting,etc

e)Exposure to cellphones,TV,Computers,chemicals that you inhale,etc

Our bodies are repairing themselves 24/7 but we are interfering with its healing process by stressing the body out ans slowing down the self healing of the body. The more stress you have in your life the sicker you will be and the less stress you have in your life the healthier you're gonna be. You should always be calm in any situation and to eliminate all stress from your life and if that's not possible for you then you should reduce it as much as you can. Eliminating or reducing all your stress is not gonna happen over night,it will take time or a lot of time depending on how much stress you have in your life. Stress=Health problems and a lot of stress will cause disease or kill you. Here are the people who cause the most stress in your life:

a)Your boss
b)Your medical doctor
c)Your job
d)Your mother
e)Your father
f)Your boyfriend or husband
g)Your girlfriend,fiancee or wife
h)Your children
i)Your relatives
j)Your lawyer
k)Your loser friends,etc

Note:Eliminating the stress from your life or all the stress from your life is NOT gonna happen overnight. It could take months or even years to live a stress free life.
You need to be patient and eliminate the stress from your life little by little or if you a fast a safe way to eliminate all the stress from your life,then use it!

2-HOW TO ELIMINATE THE DEAD FOODS AND BEVERAGES FROM YOUR DIET or MINIMIZE THEM

I will now tell you a major health secret about our diet:
There are 2 types of foods:
Live foods and Dead foods
Live foods are alkaline foods and dead foods are acidic foods. Alkaline foods keep you healthy and young looking while acidic foods cause health problems,suffering,premature aging and death.
Here are a few examples of dead foods or acidic foods:
Meat,Dairy,Bread,Eggs,Fish,Flour,Pasta,Sugar,Butter,etc
All cooked foods (fried,broiled,boiled,roasted,etc)
Here are a few examples of live foods or alkaline foods:
Pumpkin,Almonds,Apples,Apricots,Oranges,Bananas,
Beets,Papaya,Cabbage,Blackberries,Blueberries,Melons,

Mango,Lemons,Raspberries,Broccoli,Cherries,
Cantaloupe,Carrots,Celery,Currants,Coconut,Cranberries,
Grapes,Grapefruit,Guava,etc.
Almost everything we eat nowadays is acidic and that's
why the health of the world is worse than ever. We
should eat a diet that is 90% alkaline and 10% acidic but
unfortunately we are doing exactly the opposite:we are
eating a diet that is 90% acidic and 10% alkaline. That's
why we have a major health crisis right now and diseases
like heart disease,cancer,stroke,diabetes,obesity,high
blood pressure,etc are on the rise.
Here's another major secret about our beverages:
There are 2 types of beverages: acidic and alkaline.
Acidic beverages make you sick
and
Alkaline beverages make you healthy
Here are a few examples of acidic beverages:
a)All bottled water(the brand doesn't matter)
b)Sodas
c)Alcohol
d)Coffee
e)Milk
f)Black tea
There are only three types of beverages that are alkaline:
a-Alkaline water
There is a saying that most people ignore but you
shouldn't,if you care about your health:
"You are what you eat"
It's 50% true because what you drink matters too.
If you eat acidic foods your body will become acidic or
sick and if you eat alkaline foods your body will become
alkaline or healthy.
"Perfect health is perfectly simple"

An alkaline body is a healthy body and an acidic body is a sick body.

You are what you eat is a very good saying but I got one that's better:

"You are what you drink"

The first and the most important thing you need to do to make your body alkaline is to drink alkaline water.

Remember that 70% of your body is water. And 80% of your brain is water. And 90% of your blood is water.

"Water is the most important ingredient for health"

And the only water that is good for your body and brain is alkaline water. Any other water is very bad for you.

Also,it is very important that you drink enough alkaline water every day. How much water should you drink daily?That depends on your weight:

If you weigh 100 lbs you should drink 50 oz of water.
If you weigh 200 lbs you should drink 100 oz of water.
If you weigh 300 lbs you should drink 150 oz of water.

In other words,you need to drink half of your body weight of water in ounces.

I did a lot of research about the best alkaline water and Kangen water is the best alkaline water in the world.

That doesn't mean that it is the best for you,too. We are all different and you might like a different type of alkaline water. Talk to an expert here about which alkaline water is right for you:

www.waterionizerexpert.com

Japan is the healthiest country in the world! Why?

Reason#1:

They drink alkaline water

Reason#2

Their diet is mostly alkaline

Reason#3

Japanese doctors heal you when you are sick unlike American doctors and many other doctors from many other countries which only treat your symptoms with poisons like:drugs,vaccines and they also mutilate your body and they call it surgery.

PS:You can drink the kangen water for free for up to a month from a kangen water independent distributor in your area or you can drink it for free directly from the company if they have an office near you. Call them an find out. Their phone number is on their website: www.enagic.com

b-The freshly squeezed juice of organic alkaline fruits and vegetables.

c-Super juices like:

Aloe vera juice

Noni juice

Goji Juice

Mangosteen juice

Monavie juice

Pomegranate juice

Blueberry juice

Cranberry juice

Cherry juice

Nopalea juice

etc

3-HOW TO CORRECT THE DEFICIENCIES IN YOUR BODY BY GIVING YOUR BODY WHAT IT NEEDS

Before I tell you how to correct the deficiencies in your body I have to tell you some important facts.

Scientists trace diseases and ailments to mineral deficiency.

Six decades ago as part of an investigation into American farming practices,a Senate Document revealed:"foods

grown on millions of acres of land no longer contain enough minerals and are starving us."Quietly hidden from the public all these decades,
this alarming study also found that 99% of North Americans had serious nutritional deficiencies. Today,modern agricultural methods have virtually eliminated nature's most important nutrient delivery carrier, fulvic acid,which helps transport more minerals,enzymes and oxygen to the cells and the result is millions of people with chronic diseases.
Two times Nobel Laureate,Dr Paul Linus,said: "You could trace every disease and every ailment to a mineral deficiency."Approximately 99% of the human body is comprised of minerals,yet minerals are generally overlooked when nutrition is considered. It is well known that the human body requires at least 70 minerals in order to maintain a disease and ailment free state.
Thanks to this important information,it's now easy to understand why sickness is so widespread throughout the world,even in technologically advanced countries.
Fact:
The body can utilize minerals without vitamins but it cannot utilize vitamins without minerals
The foods we raise or purchase in markets today,seldom contain more than 18 to 20 minerals.
This small number of minerals in plants is because of a mineral deficiency of the food producing soils around the world. This is caused by thousands of years of erosion,fertilizers,air and water pollution and unethical farming practices. Except for nitrogen,phosphorus and potassium,the agriculture industry doesn't replenish minerals depleted from the soils. Ironically,these three are the primary ones required to grow beautiful plants

and produce but do not provide all that our bodies require. Extensive research is showing that without supplementation,it is not likely that we can eat enough food to get the full range of essential trace minerals required to obtain optimum health and live a long life free of disease. Research has also found that without the proper nutrients,our cells experience a breakdown that can lead to degenerative diseases. Decades of pesticides,herbicides,toxins and pollution have drained our farmlands and food supply of their vital elements including organic fulvic acid,a natural molecule long considered one of the most complete answers to the body's need for life-giving minerals,oxygen,enzymes and amino acids. In other words,if you eat just food,it's not enough. You have to supplement your body with:vitamins,minerals,herbs,amino-acids,fiber,carbohydrates,proteins,fats,etc.

So,what does your body need? Quality Nutrition!

"If you eat just food,that is not good"

There are many wonderful nutrition products out there that will significantly improve your health or help give you perfect health but you are not gonna find them in stores. The nutrition products that are sold in supermarkets are good......good for nothing that is!

They are useless or they will make a little or no difference in your health. The nutrition products that are sold in vitamin shops are a little better.

Still,you can take them forever and it will not improve your health significantly. Products that will help your body eliminate any health problem you have are not sold in any store in the world. They are sold by nutrition network marketing companies or nutrition MLM companies. So,what is the right nutrition program for you?

When it comes to nutrition one nutrition program doesn't fit all so find a MLM nutrition company that you like best from the internet,use their amazing unique products that work and start to look and feel better in 30 days or less. Some people feel the difference in just a few hours. I know I did!Everybody is different but you will definitely improve your health and eventually eliminate all your health problems that are keeping you from enjoying life. Also,you can email me and I'll tell you which MLM nutrition program is right for you!

There is a formula for good health:

"Good nutrition=Good Health"

Here's my version of that formula:

"Perfect Nutrition=Perfect Health"

However,it takes more than perfect nutrition to have perfect health. I'll tell you more about that soon!

PS:Since I've been using nutrition products from MLM nutrition companies,I have had amazing health benefits:

1-Unlimited energy 24/7

(I simply forgot how it feels to be tired anymore!)

2-I do not get colds anymore

3-I don't get sick anymore and all my health problems have disappeared forever!

HOW TO ENJOY PERFECT HEALTH FOREVER

Fact:

70% of diseases are diet related diseases

That means that most of what you eat and drink daily is either making you sick or keeping you healthy.

Where does your health come from?

70%=your diet---20%=your stress---10%=your genes

Hippocrates (460B.C.-377 B.C.),a Greek doctor said:

"Our food should be our medicine.
Our medicine should be our food"
Coincidentally there are two things you have to do to
have perfect health forever and perfect health has two
words,also!
Here are the 2 things you must do to enjoy perfect health
forever:
1-Give your body what it needs
2-Don't give your body what it doesn't need
My mind invented this saying about the body:
"If you give your body what it needs,your body will give
you what you need"
And what do you need?
Perfect health!
1-Here's what you need to have in your life to enjoy
perfect health forever:
1-Pure air
2-Pure water
3-Natural toothpaste,soap,shampoo,conditioner,detergent,
dish washing liquid,hair color,etc
4-The right nutrition program
5-Organic food
6-The right amount of sunlight
7-The right amount of money
8-The right amount of rest
9-The right amount of exercise
10-The right amount of friends
11-The right amount of sex
12-The right doctor which can only be a natural doctor
13-A shower filter
14-A house filter
15-Keeping your body free of toxins

2-Here's what you don't need to have in your life to enjoy perfect health forever:

1-People that could ruin your health like:
a)Regular medical doctors or M.D.'s
b)Bosses
c)Drug users
d)Boozers
e)Liars
f)Pessimists
g)Negative people
h)Complainers
i)Racists
j)Morons
k)Verbal fights
l)A romantic relationship

2-Poisons like:
a)Prescription drugs or legal drugs
b)Illegal drugs
c)Vaccines
d)Tobacco
e)Alcohol
f)Coffee
g)Milk
h)Tea
i)Bottled Water
j)Sodas
k)Sugar
l)Microwaved foods
m)Meat
n)Foods that your body is allergic to
o)Stress
p)Amalgam fillings

1-Give your body what it needs

1-Pure air

If you are living near the beach or the mountains or in a city where your air is pure then you got nothing to worry about. If you live in a city that has dirty air then purify that air immediately!I dare you! And make sure you purify the air for the entire city so everybody can breathe clean healthy air! There is nothing you can do about the dirty outdoors air except complain about it but these is something you can do about the air inside your apartment or home.

Buy an air purifier and breathe pure air every day and you will significantly improve your health.

I did a lot of research and I recommend you buy an air filter from here:

http://www.alpineairtechnologies.com

2-Pure water

There is only one water that you need to drink and it's called":

"ALKALINE WATER"

This water has been called:"The fountain of youth".If you are drinking bottled water,no matter the brand,you are making yourself sick slowly but surely.

Fact:

"B.W. is B.W."

The first B.W. stands for Bottled Water and the second B.W. stands for Bullshit Water!

All bottled water is bullshit water

It doesn't matter what company makes it,it has been proved scientifically that bottled water is bad for you for more than one reason:high on chemicals,low on minerals,etc and it's acidic meaning it makes you sick,slowly but surely.

PS:Alkaline water is so good for your body that you can even lose weight on it. I myself lost 10lbs in 30 days! This live miraculous water is a must for you if you want perfect health and on the internet you can see many health testimonials of what this healthy water did for other people.

The best alkaline water that I found so far is here: www.ameritek.net or www.puronics.com

3-Natural toothpaste,natural shaving cream,natural soap,natural shampoo and conditioner,natural detergent,natural deodorant,natural dish washing liquid,natural hair color, natural hair spray,etc

You should use only organic or natural toothpaste,soap,shampoo,conditioner,detergent,dish washing liquid,hair color,etc because the ones that are sold in stores are harmful to your health. They are loaded with chemicals that cause serious health problems like cancer mostly. The skin that is like a sponge and it absorbs anything you put on it. For example: every time you use a toothpaste that is not organic or natural,the chemicals from that toothpaste will get absorbed into your blood stream and over time can do some damage to you health. Every time you use a shampoo or a shaving cream that is not organic or natural you are putting your health in danger.

Have you noticed lately that breast cancer is on the rise? Why do you think that is? I'll tell you why:because women are using non-organic or not natural deodorants that are toxic and those toxins get absorbed into the bloodstream and over time they get to the breasts and breast cancer is the result. Stay way from any non-organic or not natural personal care products including your detergent you use to wash your clothes. Why?

Because the clothes you just washed with a non-organic or not natural detergent are full of harmful chemicals and your skin will absorb them and over time will cause health problems or disease.

4-The right nutrition program

Here's another lie:"If one eats a healthy diet,one does not need any supplementation" Fact:

"One has to supplement their diet in order to give the body all the nutrition it needs on a daily basis"

An American doctor said something interesting:

"It is not what you eat that kills you,it is what you don't eat that kills you"

He is right but not 100% right. He is only 50% right. It is what you eat that kills you also. What's wrong with today's food? It is deficient in nutrients and it is high in p poisons that are making you sick. There are many poisons in our foods like chemicals,MSG,additives, artificial coloring,hormones,antibiotics,pesticides,etc. Avoid all these poisons if you want to keep enjoying your perfect health. These are just 10 poisons they add to our foods to prolong shelf life. They don't care about our health,they only care about their profits.

There are many more poisons out there. I suggest you read the labels of every grocery you buy and if you see something that you don't recognize,then most likely it's bad for your body. If you wanna know more about the non-organic foods that you eat every day and if you wanna know more about how they are grossly mistreating the animals and the farmers,I suggest watching these informative movies:

a)Food matters

b)Food,inc

c)Fast food nation

5-Organic food

If should eat only organic food or clean food if you wanna be healthy. If you eat non-organic food or dirty food,you are not eating just food,you are also putting in your your body the following harmful ingredients:chemicals,pesticides,hormones, antibiotics,etc and they will damage your health over time.Also,when you go and eat out,that is the worst food you can put in your body. Never ever eat fast food because that's the fastest way to make yourself sick or die prematurely.

I strongly recommend that you to see the documentary movie:"Supersize me" and you'll see for how deadly fast food is. After seeing the movie myself,I never walked into a fast food place ever again!Also,if you eat out,I recommend the only 2 places you can go and enjoy clean and healthy food:restaurants that sell raw food organic food.Let me throw you a bone here:

"Bone" "app-eh-tit"!

6-The right amount of sunlight:

Here is another major lie I'm gonna expose:

Lie:

"Use sunscreen to prevent skin cancer"

Truth:

"Sunscreen doesn't prevent skin cancer,it causes it"

Getting a lot of sun will never give you skin cancer and you need at least 15 minutes of sun every day in order to have perfect health. Me and all my family and friends have been in the sun every day of our lives for the last 40 years and we never got skin cancer and we never will. If the sun caused skin cancer then everybody in Africa should have skin cancer right? But you know that's not the case here. Here's what really causes skin cancer:the sunscreen products you put on your face to "protect" you from the sun because they are loaded with dangerous chemicals and they are absorbed by the skin and the result is skin cancer.

WARNING:

"Do not ever use sunscreen that has chemicals in it"
If you do,don't be surprised if you get skin cancer.

7-The right amount of money

Here is another lie:"Money doesn't bring happiness"
Truth:"Money brings a lot of happiness and the more money you have the happier you are"
99% of the people in this world are broke or worse:they are over-broke or they are in debt. Can you be broke and happy? I don't think so. You can solve virtually every problem you have if you had enough money.

Here are a few examples:

a)If you won the lottery of let's say 10 million dollars,that wouldn't make you happy? You can go on a shopping spree and buy whatever your heart desires.
I believe that shopping makes everybody happy, don't you stink,I mean think?

b)The number one problem humanity has right now is health. We are having a major health crisis right now. Humanity has never suffered like this because of health problems in all history of mankind.
How many people do you know that are happy with the way they look and the way they feel every day? Probably none!Most people have health problems and many people have a long list of health problems. How do you solve these problems? Money! And lots of it because you're gonna need to see a natural doctor and he or she ain't cheap and your health insurance,if you have one,does not cover natural doctors. Fortunately the stuff I'm taking:the

best nutrition program and the best drink in the world can be afforded by virtually anybody.

c)The fights between parents and their children can be avoided if the kids had enough money to move out and live a peaceful and happy life.

d)Why are most people struggling to pay their bills every month? Because they don't have enough money. If they did,the struggle will over forever.

e)If you are a parent and you have kids,why can't you buy your kids whatever they want? Because you don't have enough money. If you did,then you can take your kids shopping and buy them whatever they want.

f)Why can't many people go to college or a university and get a good education? Because they don't have enough money. If they did,they can go to any college or university they choose.

g)Why can't people buy the car and house of their dreams? Because they don't have enough money.

h)When people have legal problems can they afford a good lawyer? No way. They are way too expensive and most people get a public defendant because they don't have enough money.

i)Most people think they are free but they aren't. They are actually in jail. They are in a financial jail. There is so much happiness out there but most people can't afford it because the best things out there are also the most expensive. For example:a really fine car would be a Lamborghini Diablo but how many people can afford $250,000? to buy it? Very few. So how do you solve your money problems once and forever? There are many ways to go from rags to riches but here is my favorite one:

Start your own home based business and make as much money as you like. If you don't know which is a good home based business to start from home for about $100,e-mail me and I'll tell you which home based business opportunity I found and I am doing. I call it the most exciting and the most fun biz opp I have ever found and it wasn't easy finding it. I literally looked at hundreds if not thousands of money making opportunities and my search is finally over. Fact:

In this world 99% of people work for the 1%

Which do ya wanna be? The broke 99% or the rich 1%?

8-The right amount of rest

Everybody is different so the right amount of sleep will vary from person to person. Too much sleep cannot hurt you but too little sleep can. I slept 15 hours a night for 20 years when I was severely depressed and I still enjoy perfect health today and now I sleep 8-10 hours a night,sometimes more but never less!

You should get a minimum of 6-8 hours of sleep every night if you wanna have perfect health.

Some of you will need more than 8 hours of sleep. "You will always need more sleep many times but you'll never need less sleep"

When I say more sleep,I'm talking about more than 8 hours of sleep and when I say less sleep,I am talking about more than 8 hours of sleep.

While you are sleeping your body is repairing itself and if you don't get enough sleep for whatever reason your body is not gonna have the time to heal itself and over time you will get sick. Do you want perfect health? Then give your body the perfect amount of sleep every night!

9-The right amount of exercise

The right amount of exercise will be different for everybody. Too much exercise can hurt you and too little exercise can also hurt you. How much exercise is the right amount? The right amount of exercise is daily exercise and it doesn't matter what kind of exercise it is. Walking is the best form of exercise they say and they could be right. The body was made for movement and if you don't move it daily then don't expect to enjoy perfect health forever. The perfect amount of exercise is different for everybody so only you know how much exercise is right for you. Nobody knows your body better than you,right? There is something better than exercise:Sex! Sex feels great,right? Yes it does,if you ever felt it before! What do you get if you com,com,combine sex and exercise? Yes,I stuttered on purpose! Sex+Exercise=Sexercise! So you should also sexercise because you get your exercise and your pleasure! WARNING:Too much exercise is bad for you and it could make you sick or kill you. Too little exercise is bad for you but it won't kill you. However it may cause a lot of health problems. And a lot of sex may cause a lot of pleasure! Attention men:Say this to a woman: "It's a pleasure to pleasure you" PS:There is no such thing as too much sex! Have at it! 10-The right amount of friends I suggest you remember these 3 brilliant sayings I invented about friends if you wanna be happy forever: a)"The most important people in your life are your friends" b)"The more friends you have the happier you are" c)"The best things in life are free and you get them from your friends"

The wrong friends are dangerous to your health. Make sure you befriend only winners. No losers!Here's my number one favorite saying I invented:

"Lose the losers"

What do you think about this saying:

"A stranger is a friend you haven't met yet"?

I like it too,stranger!

11-The right amount of sex

How much is the right amount of sex? The more the better! There is no such thing as too much sex,so I suggest that you have sex with as many people as you can. If you are in a closed relationship with your girlfriend or wife,then I suggest you guys become swingers! It is a lifestyle that is becoming very popular nowadays! How do I know that? Because me and my nonexistent girlfriend or wife are swingers!

Also,you should live all your sexual fantasies no matter how many you have. Guess how many sexual fantasies I have? Literally an infinite! A lousy sex life or a sexless life can damage your health. Sex feels good and it's good for your health. If you want perfect health,you have to have a perfect sex life!And if you don't know how,have no fear,the sex expert or the "sexpert" is here.

Email me and I'll show you how. Do it or do me!

12-A good natural doctor

(iridologist, naturopathic,homeopathic,acupuncturist,etc)

If you wanna keep yourself in perfect health see only natural doctors. Natural doctors cure you while medical doctors only treat your symptoms with dangerous and deadly drugs or worse:they perform surgery on your body which is never necessary except for when you get into a bad car accident,plane crash,etc. There is always a natural alternative to any surgery. Thomas Edison said: "The doctor of the future will give no medicine but will interest his patients in the care of the human frame,in diet and in the cause and prevention of disease."

13-A shower filter

Did you know that every time you take a shower you are actually drinking a glass of chlorine which is a deadly chemical? Here's how this is happening:If you don't use a shower filter,the shower water has a chlorine in it and every time you take a shower your skin absorbs some of the water and that's how chlorine gets in your body and can cause serious health problems in time.

To keep yourself healthy I suggest that you buy and use a shower filter forever. Enjoy healthy showers from now on!

14-A house filter

The need for a house water filtration system has become important due to the fact that one can no longer depend on the supply of water to be clean and most of the water supply we receive is full of chemicals including the added chemical carcinogens like chlorine and fluoride which can be very damaging to your health.

Water treatment systems or water filtration systems are a must if you want to enjoy perfect health. House water filtration systems will easily and properly eliminate the impurities of tap water so when you have to drink the water,wash your hands or take a bath,you don't have to worry about the water being dirty and you will no longer absorb the chemicals that are in the water. It is very important to invest in good water filtration equipment. Such equipment is usually not that expensive and they are really worth what you pay for them. Even if they are expensive,what's more important: The money or your health? Your health is priceless! There is an increased danger of cancer in people who take showers with chlorinated water and most tapped water today is chlorinated because most treatment facilities use chlorine to disinfect their water and protect their facilities so that they do not decay or have growth of algae,the plant that is usually found in water, because this is the most inexpensive way that they can do this. There are many types of water filtration systems on the market and most of them are effective and work well but you need to find one that will work for you. This will help you because you can then avoid such complications that come from consuming unclean water.

Such complications can be cancer,diarrhea,infections vomiting,stomach cramps,urinary tract infection and many other complications including death.

The application of a water filtration system will help minimize such hazards and will help you stay healthy.

15-Keeping your body free of toxins

There are 2 major ways to keep your body pure and healthy:

a)Fasting

b)Detoxify your body

a)You must fast at least once a year to keep your body clean. For more info go to www.fasting.com

b)Detoxify your body

There are a lot of products out there that detoxify your body but according to my research the best detoxifiers are:

1-Fasting

2-Aloe Vera Juice

3-Green Drinks

4-Chlorella

5-Spirulina

More coming soon!

What you don't need to have in your life to enjoy perfect health forever:

1-People that could ruin your health like:

a-Regular medical doctors or M.D.'s

Like I said earlier,your medical doctor can do only 2 things for you:Treat your symptoms in a barbaric way:

1)Poison you with dangerous deadly pills they call medication

2)Cut you open and tell you the surgery is needed

1)Medical doctors don't know anything about healing the body,they only know how to diagnose and treat symptoms with highly toxic,dangerous,unsafe and many times deadly pills they call medication.

If you have to see a doctor I suggest you see a natural doctor,one that will heal you,not treat you. So here's what I suggest you do when it comes to your M.D.:You should definitely "sea" your medical doctor meaning putting him under the sea!Not literally of course,but you should definitely fire him because there is only 2 horrible things he can do for you and he does it legally:

1-Your medical doctor will poison you legally

2-Your medical doctor will stick a knife in you legally

1:"Your medical doctor will poison you legally" means he will give you drugs and call it medication and tell you that you need your medication because it's good for you but I tell you that he is lying to you big time. Ready for another secret? Good!"

All prescription drugs are poison and should never be taken under any circumstances"

Exception:If you have a heart attack,an asthma attack,a panic attack,etc or your life is in danger because of injuries caused by a car accident or any accident,then it's okay to take drugs because they could save your life.

All drugs are deadly chemicals and they don't benefit the body in any way. As soon as you swallow a drug and it gets into the bloodstream,your body immediately will eliminate it as fast as possible because it's poison and has no use for it. Try this experiment at home:take any pill and put it on your tongue and see how long you can bear its disgusting taste. Do not swallow the pill because you could have serious side effects or die from it. Spit it out as soon as possible. If you put something edible in your mouth,it tastes good,you will chew it and swallow it. Example:A candy in the shape of a tablet like M&M's. If you take actual poison like cyanide and put it on your tongue your body will spit it out immediately because it's poison. Warning:Do not try this at home ever. Same thing is happening here. Here we have another evil medical illusion. The illusion is:

FICTION:"Drugs make you feel better"

Drugs do not furnish any nutrients. They have no intelligence to create new cells and repair damaged tissue. Here's how the illusion works:

You have "whatever" symptoms and you go and see your medical doctor,he or she gives you some drugs and you feel better. Did you feel better because of the drugs? No. Absolutely not. It was the perfect illusion. How can poison make you feel better? Here's how:When you take the drugs,they create the illusion of making you feel better because they paralyze your nerves and suspend vital action in your body,thus suppressing whatever symptoms are bothering you. After taking the drugs your

symptoms are gone and that's why you believe that it was the drugs that made you feel better and your health is better. In reality,your health is worse than before because drugs are chemicals that stay in your body for years and they affect the function of almost all your organs.
Drugs are dead and deadly and they should never ever be introduced into your body which is alive.
Here's another big health secret:
"There was never a drug that cured anything and there will never be one"
If you think the story that a vaccine cured polio is a true story,then think again:it didn't. Polio was a scam created in the 40's and today people still believe they cured polio! They actually created the scam "polio" and made many people sick by poisoning them with a vaccine invented by an idiot whose name I will not mention.
Lately,they came up with more scams than ever:
The flu shot
The swine flu
The avian flu
The h1n1 flu
The West Nile Virus
SARS
Legionnaire's disease
Lyme disease
Whopping cough(TDAP)
Shingles,Etc
In the future they will come up with more scams because the more scams they come up with the more money they make. Do not believe these evil deadly lies because they could kill you. Also,almost all drugs are highly addictive. If you wanna stay alive,stay away from all drugs and all vaccines. Millions of people around the world die each

year because of prescribed drugs by their own medical doctors. Check out this tragic fact:

"In the year 2009,there weren't any deaths caused by supplements. In the same year,over 100,000 people died from prescription drugs and countless people died from illness."

Many celebrities died from an overdose of prescription drugs. Here is a website where you will find 18 celebrities who died because of prescription drugs overdose:

http://www.pharmacytechs.net/blog/18-celebrities-who-died-from-prescription-drugs

On the internet you can see for yourself how dangerous and deadly presc-RIP-tion drugs are for you.

Did you know that:

"More people die each year from legal drugs than from illegal drugs"

Now you do so if you know what's good for you,you should never do legal drugs. And of course,illegal drugs.

2:"Your medical doctor will stick a knife in you legally" meaning he or she will operate on you and almost all surgeries are unnecessary. Why do they cut people open and perform surgeries on them? You should know the answer by now:money,big money.

Surgeons and hospitals are making millions of dollars doing this. Possibly billions. I'm gonna cut out the bullshit now and tell you another major health secret:

"There is an alternative to almost any surgery"

Here's an example:a woman was told by her doctor that is she doesn't have surgery for her cancer tumor she will die but this woman was like me:she doesn't want to be cut open ever. So she saw a natural doctor and he told her to fast for a month and she did. After a month of fasting she

was cancer free and her tumor was gone. I'm gonna tell you now the fastest way to perfect health:Fasting! It's possible that you do not know what that means and that's why I'll explain it. When you are fasting you are avoiding food and you are only drinking liquids like water or juice. You can do a water fast where you drink only water or a juice fast where you drink only freshly squeezed juices. Fasting has been around for ten thousand years and is the best thing you can do for your body. Nothing beats fasting and no matter if you are sick or healthy I recommend you do a fast but make sure it's supervised by a professional. Many severe diseases like cancer,diabetes,schizophrenia, depression,etc have disappeared after people fasted. It's the fastest way to eliminate virtually any health problem.
Fasting can also save your life. It definitely saved the life of one of my friends twice when she was feeling so horrible and she didn't want to live anymore because her suffering was unbearable. Fasting saved the lives of so many people and it can save yours too. In case you don't know what fasting is:To fast means to avoid all foods and drink only water or juice or both.
Fiction:
Not eating is bad for your health or it can kill you
Fact:
"Not eating food for up to 30 days is the best thing ever you can do for your health"
When you don't eat the body has a lot of extra energy to detoxify,repair and heal itself.
Warning:Never do an unsupervised fast. Always fast under the supervision of a professional fasting practitioner. Never ever fast alone.

Replace your loser medical doctor with a winner doctor aka a natural doctor. Here are some examples of natural doctors that will help your body cure itself:

1-A natural doctor(A Naturopath,A Homeopath,An acupuncturist,a Natural Hygienist,An Iridologist,etc)

2-An acupuncturist

3-An herbalist

4-An irodologist

5-A hypnotist

A doctor that will never give you pills or operate on you.A doctor who will help your body heal and not treat your symptoms.Here's a major reason to keep M.D.'s out of your life forever:

Here are the 3 major causes of death today:

1)Heart Disease

2)Cancer

3)Doctors and hospitals

I came up with a nickname for doctors:"Doctorers"

How? I combined the word doctor and murderer!

Medical doctors are killing people legally and getting away with with it. Sad but true.

b-Bosses

Your boss is causing you so much stress in your life that it could make you sick or really sick. Let me expose another lie:"Slavery was abolished over 200 years ago"

Truth:Slavery is still alive and well and 99% of us are slaves except we are not called slaves anymore,we are called employees. We are still slaves except we are modern slaves and we are actually getting paid for our work:chump change compared to the money the company we work for makes. Being an employee for whatever company is very dangerous to your health because of the following reasons:

a)You never make enough money
b)You never get enough vacation time
c)You do the same thing every day
d)You might not like your job
Fact:
Most people hate their jobs
e)Your co-workers might be bothering you,talking bad about you,hurting you,wanting your position or stalking you
f)You are under constant fear and stress that one day you might lose your job and you definitely will lose it one day
g)Your job will never make you rich,it makes the company you work for rich while keeping you broke
h)You can get seriously injured or die on the job
i)You are always told what to do when you have a job-do you like to be told what to do? Neither do I!
To avoid being a slave aka an employee you need to work for yourself and be your own boss.
c-Drug addicts
Drugs users are low life losers and you should never befriend one. Stay away from them forever. Also,drug users are criminals because they are breaking the law. There is a saying:"Winners don't do drugs" so if you are a winner you shouldn't hang out with losers aka drug users. So don't get addicted to drug addicts,get addicted to sober people!
d-Boozers
If you wanna keep your health perfect here is a perfect advise:Don't ever drink this poisonous liquid called alcohol. Keep it out of your body and keep boozers out of your life. Drunks are low life losers and you should lose them all!

Boozers are low life losers!

e-Liars

Have you ever heard the saying:

"You lie and your happiness will die"?

Of course you haven't because I invented the saying myself! To me lying is unacceptable and I ended a lot of friendships because people have lied to me.

"Honesty is the best policy" is a saying that I believe in 100% but unfortunately we all have to lie sometimes for whatever reason. Don't worry about me lying to you in my book because every frigging word I wrote is true!

Does that sound good to you?

My advise to you:Never lie to anybody unless you absolutely have to for whatever reason and then one day in the future when you are "out of the woods" you should tell that person that you lied to them and apologize.

Bingo,I just gave you the ultimate secret about how to never lie to anybody ever and feel good yourself and have a clear conscience!Liars are bad for your health because lying is like a disease and you might "catch" it from them and become a liar yourself! So,stay away from liars because they are a waste of your precious time!

Do you think I'm lying to you?

Maybe!

Maybe not! Maybe nut! Am I nuts? Nuts anyone?

f-Pessimists

There are 2 types of people in this world:

1)Winners

2)Losers

99% of people on this planet are losers and 1% are winners. Pessimists are definitely losers because when they look at the future they see a negative,unhappy future

If you have pessimists in your life get rid of them

immediately because they can affect your health severely.

Here's an example:Let's say you have terminal cancer,right? A pessimist like your M.D. will tell you that you have 6 to 9 months to live. An optimist like a natural doctor will tell you that you're not gonna die and he will heal you also.

Fiction:"Terminal diseases will kill you in a few months"

Fact:

"Almost all terminal diseases can be cured if you fast or go to the right natural doctor"

Pessimists do not see perfect health in your future so stay away from them like you stay away from the news on TV which are mostly negative.

g-Negative people

When you are 100% positive that a person is negative,make sure that:

1)If they are already your friends,dump them faster than you dumped yesterday's newspaper

2)If they are not your friends and they are strangers,make sure they stay that way

Here's another saying I invented:"Danger starts with a stranger".Also,you should never be or think negative because it is literally bad for your health.

So,if you wanna have perfect health,the first thing you have to do is believe that it is possible for you and it is and the second thing is think like this:I will have perfect health,it is just a matter of time!

h)Complainers

Here's a saying that an intelligent self made millionaire friend of mine invented:

"You can't complain. Who are you to complain to anybody about anything?"

Complaining about anything doesn't solve any problems and it only accomplishes 2 things:
1-You're wasting your time
2-You are wasting your breath
Never complain about anything or anybody because you just wasted precious energy that the body can use to heal itself. If you must complain,do it in your mind and make it as short as possible. Remember that your body has limited energy to heal itself and when you complain you are not letting the body do its job. The more you complain the more damage you are doing to your body. Don't complain about complainers,keep them out of your life and keep enjoying perfect health!

i)Racists

Racists are people that hate certain races of people. Did you know that hating anything or anybody is bad for your health? Here's what good for your health:Love! It's never OK to be a racist because there is only one race out there:The human race. If you are a racist and if you want to have perfect health,keep dreaming. It's not gonna happen. If you have friends that are racists then I suggest you make an exception and become a racist yourself meaning:Be a racist against only one race:The racists!In other words,racist are bad for your health and I suggest you start believing in E-racism!
Erase all your racists from your life forever and erase any health problems they might cause you!

j)Morons

Morons are bad for your health. If you have any health problems and don't know what to do,they can give you stupid advice like:"Go ask your medical doctor" and that is very dangerous to your health!Don't ever listen to stupid people's advise. However,I agree with one thing here:I suggest you go and ask,I mean "axe" your medical doctor! Not literally of course but you should fire your medical doctor and hire a natural doctor.

Now that's smart advise coming from a genius like me who speaks 5 more languages fluently besides English! So,don't be stupid and don't befriend stupid people,either! Befriend smart people like me!

PS:Besides English I speak: Romanian,Macedonian,Spanish,French and Italian. I'm still learning many other languages. I am also a language freak!

k)Verbal fights

Verbal fights are interfering with the body's healing process. Every time you fight you are making your body acidic or sick so do not fight with anybody for any reason if you want perfect health.

l)A romantic relationship

Do you think that the future can be predicted with 100% accuracy? I agree with you!I'm gonna predict something right now that is 100% accurate. Here it is:"Not everybody will agree with what I'm about to say about romantic relationships" See? I told you I can predict the future with 100% accuracy!Have you ever heard the saying:"Happiness is being single"?I did and I believe it's 100% true but it might not be true for you.

Most people get married and have kids and then you have the rest of us who like to stay single forever and have no kids. I am single with no kids,I always was and I always will be. Why? Because that's what makes me happy. I will never have a girlfriend,a wife or kids and I do that to keep my perfect health perfect. Having a girlfriend,boyfriend,husband or wife can be very dangerous to your health. Here's why. He or she might:

1)murder you(worst case scenario)
2)cheat on you
3)break your heart
4)control your life
5)ruin your sex life
6)verbally abuse you
7)ruin you financially
8)physically abuse you
9)dump you for somebody else
10)give you an STD!Just kidding!
Actually they can give you an STD that actually exists and it's the worst possible "STD"you can get:they can give you a kid or worse:kids!Now,that is an STD that could ruin your happiness forever and ever and ever! There's no happily ever after here!
Let's see why:
1)Kids are very expensive to raise
2)They can be born retarded or with a serious physical defect
3)They can be born dead
4)They can be born evil
5)They might hate you instead of loving you
6)They might murder you
7)They might die young and you'll suffer forever
8)They might wanna marry somebody you don't like
9)They might fight with you verbally or physically,etc
So,if you wanna maintain your perfect health I suggest you avoid these 3 "poisons":
1-Girlfriend or Boyfriend
2-Wife or Husband
3-Kids or adopted kids
Please note that I said "I suggest" meaning you don't have to take my advise. You do whatever you want

because you have free will. Sometimes you have to learn a lesson in life the hard way. Not only do I invent my own sayings but I also improve existing sayings.
The saying:"Happiness is being single" was improved by me and here is my version:
"Happiness is being single,healthy and wealthy"
Here's another saying I invented about relationships:
"Closed-minded people have closed relationships and open-minded people have open relationships"
I am single and happy and I plan to keep it that way until the day I pass away and I don't believe in any relationships but if you must have one have an open relationship because it lasts longer and it's good for your health. Having a closed relationship lasts shorter and it's bad for your health. Finally,no matter if you have a closed or open relationship,when you are in a relation with someone you are giving up a percentage of your freedom and being free is one of the ingredients of perfect health.
2-Poisons like:
a)Legal drugs or prescription drugs
Pills kill millions of people around the world every day. They are literally chemicals or poisons and they should never ever be taken because they cause disease,suffering and death. Here is a saying a brilliant natural doctor invented:
"The best medicine is no medicine"
Here is some wise advise from a very wise man from a long time ago:
"Nearly all men die of their medicines,not of their diseases."
Did this guy know something we don't know today?

Yes he did and now you know too!Say good bye to imperfect medicine and say hello to perfect health!
b)Illegal drugs or recreational drugs
Illegal drugs or recreational drugs are addictive and bad to your health. Do you know how much damage they can do to you? They will damage you permanently and if you don't stop taking them they could end your life.
You know that saying:"You don't do drugs,drugs do you"? It's 100% true! The best thing to do is to never start taking drugs because they are illegal first of all and if you take them that makes you a criminal. Besides putting your health and life in danger you are also putting your freedom in danger:You do the crime,you do the time. Keep deadly illegal drugs outside your life and keep your body pure and healthy on the inside!
c)Vaccines
Here are another 2 double deadly global lies:
"Vacciness prevent disease"
and
"Vaccines eliminated a lot of diseases"
Fact:
"Vaccines cause disease and death. Vaccines cause autism,paralysis,etc. Never ever vaccinate yourself because if you do the consequences are devastating"

Here's another deadly global lie against our pets:
"Vaccinate your pets against rabies"
Fact:
Rabies is a scam
it doesn't exist so if you love your pets never ever give them any vaccines. The ingredients in almost all vaccines are the deadliest poisons you can ever imagine like:

Formaldehyde,Aspartame,Mercury,Mono-sodium glutamate (MSG),Phosphate,Bacterial Waste, Aluminum potassium sulfate,Aluminum,Antibiotics, Hydroxyde, Thimerosal,Glycerin,Phenol, Sorbitol, Phenoxyethenol, Cancerous Cells,Feces,Urine,etc.
Yuck,that's gross and disgusting.
I call that:"Dis-gross-ting"!
Do not ever vaccinate yourself,your kids or your pets,EVER.
Fact:
Vaccines cause disease,they don't prevent it
Vaccines cause many horrible diseases and death.
Diseases like measles,mumps,chicken pox,etc. But what did they tell us about the above diseases? They told us that those diseases have disappeared thanks to vaccines. So they are telling us that vaccines cure diseases. Really? I'm not convinced!
"The sad truth is that no vaccine has ever eradicated any disease and no vaccine ever will"
These evil bastards are monsters. They tell us these deadly evil lies who destroy families and make millions of innocent people suffer needlessly and die.
Who cares about the people,right? As long as these greedy evil heartless soulless demons make billions of dollars in profit.
Vaccines also cause other horrible diseases like:diabetes, lung cancer,epilepsy,polio, asthma,rubella,brain damage, nervous system malfunction, anaphylactic shock(extreme allergic reaction),arthritis, Alzheimer's disease,cancer,etc.
It gets worse:vaccines also killed millions of babies worldwide and unfortunately it's still happening today.
When babies would die from Shaken baby syndrome they blamed it on many innocent parents who were

arrested and charged with the crime of killing their newborn children in violent attempts to get them to stop crying and go back to sleep. When babies died of crib death-also known as sudden infant death syndrome or SIDS,they couldn't blame that on anybody or anything because they didn't know what killed these precious poor newborn babies. Now educated people like me and you know the real cause for The shaken baby syndrome and SIDS:(Sudden Infant Death Syndrome):Vaccines Vaccines:they are the cause for the baby genocide. Here's how this deadly evil scam works: According to them inoculations or vaccinations work on the premise that our bodies will create antibodies to the pathogens (deadly toxins) found within the vaccines. If we have antibodies,we are immune to the particular disease in question. If we are immune,we can't catch disease. This theory of theirs sounds very convincing but what about AIDS? With most other diseases,if you have the antibodies to that disease,you cannot catch the disease because you are immune to the disease but with AIDS,if you have the antibodies to HIV, you are said to be HIV-positive and at risk for AIDS.
This is also the case with all other viral diseases.

Since no one can find a virus (which is a blatant violation of Koch's postulates,one of the cornerstones of the contagion theory),the only way to detect a virus is to detect its antibodies. But if we have antibodies,we're immune!That's the whole premise of immunization. So,on the one hand,if you have antibodies,you have immunity but on the other hand,if you have antibodies you are at risk. These murderous idiots are contradicting themselves. They tell us two contradicting stories and they tell us they are both true stories. That's like saying:The milk is white-true story. The milk is black-also true story. They may have fooled virtually everybody on this planet but not me. And you my precious reader now know the truth and they can't fool you anymore. Even more important,they cannot poison you legally and make you really sick or worse:kill you with their deadly legal poison they call:Vaccines.

Vaccinated=Terminated

To get vaccinated means to poison your blood which means expect disease,suffering and premature death. Again,the body is very simple in operation. If you drink or eat something that it cannot use,your body immediately tries to get rid of it. The more toxins you give your body,the more your body tries to eliminate them but there comes a time when these toxins are stored in the cells of your body for too long.

The normal channels of elimination such as defecation,urination, respiration and perspiration are enough to eliminate all toxic substances from the body but when toxins are stored for prolonged periods of time,they must be eliminated through alternate channels and that is why you develop symptoms such as irritability,fatigue,drowsiness,nausea,diarrhea, constipation,vomiting,bloating,fever,headaches,trouble sleeping,nightmares,nasal drip,coughing, sneezing, pustules,boils,skin breakouts,acne,congestion,flu like symptoms,pain,etc.

Detoxify or die

And it's not gonna be a quick painless death. It's gonna be a long(years or decades) slow agonizing painful death. Your body uses these alternate channels for the purposes of detoxification but according to them,what are you

supposed to do when you develop such symptoms? You are supposed to take medications(more toxins)to relieve yourself of these symptoms. How moronic!So if you listen to them,you stop the detoxification, which forces your body to restore the toxins,thus setting you up for a more difficult detoxification in the future and if you never detoxify your body,then expect some major suffering in your future or an early death.
If you want perfect health,then you better do the perfect detox which is a yearly detox!

d)Tobacco

As you already know almost half a million Americans die from smoking each year and before you die from cigarettes you will get a lot of health problems from smoking like:cancer,emphysema,ED(erectile dysfunction),bad breath,yellow teeth,etc. You should never smoke cigarettes or cigars,never chew any tobacco and if you are doing it then stop before your health goes up in smoke! It's easier than ever nowadays to quit smoking especially with the introduction of electrical cigarettes which will satisfy your craving for smoking but they are harmless. If you wanna live or achieve perfect health,then say no...to... to-bac-co!
Ho,ho,hoes!

e)Alcohol

All alcohol is poison and you should never drink it because its side effects are many. Here are a few:
1)Alcohol is expensive for most people
2)Alcohol is addictive and it may ruin your life
3)Alcohol is acidic and it may age you faster
4)Alcohol can damage or destroy your liver
5)Alcohol can cause many health problems and it may make your stomach fat

6)Alcohol can severely impair your judgment
7)Alcohol in excess makes you drunk and you may be raped,you may drive drunk and kill yourself or other people or both,you might get violent and get into physical fights and you might commit murder when drunk and not even realize it.

Here's another lie."Wine in small amounts every day is good for your heart health".Fact:Wine in any amounts is still poison and bad for your health.

Fact:

"They lie so you can buy"
But I tell you not to buy....this lie!

f)Coffee

First of all,coffee contains a ton of caffeine. Caffeine is addictive and it could be a drug and comes with an extended list of bad side effects. The headache that comes on when you are trying to kick this unhealthy habit will be brutal and creating a dependency and addiction like this is often harmful to the body.

Second,coffee is extraordinarily acidic.

Our bodies perform at optimum levels once they are slightly alkaline (the opposite of acidic).An acidic body's pH is like a magnet for all kinds of illnesses. Additionally,an alkaline body features an abundant stronger immune system, creating illness much less likely. Last however not least,the caffeine in coffee is abuse to your adrenal glands. Your adrenals release your "fight or flight" hormones essentially supplying you with a nice "boost" when needed. Unfortunately,individuals who drink occasional all day long are consistently beating on their adrenals. This is often the equivalent of whipping a tired horse even when he's exhausted. Eventually he will not move at all. If you ever heard that you will have any health benefits from drinking coffee don't believe it because it comes from the ones who make billions of dollars selling coffee and it's another global lie. Eliminate this poison from your life before it eliminates the life from you!Just like the alcohol and tobacco industry,the coffee industry also makes billions of dollars so of course they are gonna tell you that coffee is good for you. Coffee is bad for you and do not ever tell this to anybody ever again:Do you wanna go out for a coffee unless you are trying to poison them! Would you like some coffee? If your answer is yes then coffee can help you get into an early coff-in!

PS:Every rule has an exception. Not all coffee is bad for you. Here is one of many places where you will find coffee that is good for you:
www.healthycoffeeusa.com

g)Milk

Got Milk? I hope not cuz if you do,it will do you in! Milk is one of the deadliest beverages you can drink. You should never drink milk. If you drink cow milk you will get a lot of health problems. Here is one website that tells you why milk is very dangerous to your health:
http://www.notmilk.com

h)Tea

Are you surprised if I told you that is not good for your health? You shouldn't be! Drinking tea is bad for your health:

1)Drinking tea could cause chromosome damage and fetal leukemia

2)Phytochemicals, derived from plant foods and present in tea extracts, could have biological activity in the body and cause dangerous side effects.

3)Tea-based dietary supplements causes hepatotoxicity or chemical-induced liver damage
4)Tea could damage human chromosomes,pose harm to pregnant women and increase the risk of leukemia among unborn babies. Also,research on rats and dogs found a potential for kidney and intestinal damage. Even worse,after drinking tea the mice's tiny balls got even tinier! Such a tiny mouse tragedy!
Exception:Some teas are good for you like organic teas and herbal teas. So,what would you like to drink? Coffee,milk or tea? If you answered "None of the above" then you are on your way to perfect health!
PS:Some teas are good for you like green tea or any organic tea!

i)Bottled water
Fiction:"Bottled water is good for your health"
All bottled water is diseased water. It doesn't matter what the brand is,it has been proven scientifically that bottled water is bad for you for more than one reason.
It has been proved scientifically that bottled water is bad for you because:
1)It's acidic
2)It can cause cancer
3)high on chemicals
4)low on minerals
5)It can kill you if it's contaminated (Almost 1,000,000 people die yearly because of contaminated water!)

j)Sodas
Do you know what I call sodas?
"Cancer in a can"
After vaccines and alcohol,the most dangerous liquid you can drink is sodas. All sodas are very harmful and the two that do the most damage to your health are the 2

most popular ones. You know their names. Here's is a hint:One starts with C and the other one starts with P.

1)Sodas are very acidic (as acidic as battery acid)

2)Sodas contain sugar,a disease causing poison

3)Sodas will age you faster

4)Sodas can cause many diseases including cancer

5)Sodas can cause tooth decay

6)Sodas can cause hyperactivity

7)Sodas are addictive

8)Sodas are carbonated and that is harmful to your stomach and other organs

9)Sodas contain caffeine,calories and many harmful chemicals

10)Sodas can make you fat

If you wanna stay close to perfect health then I suggest you stay away from all sodas,all the time!

PS:Replace unhealthy drinks like alcohol,coffee,tea,sodas,etc with healthy juices like: Aloe Vera juice, Noni juice, Goji juice,Mangosteen Juice, Monavie Juice,etc and start enjoying much better health. Also, drinks that are too cold or too hot are not good for your health. Finally,all carbonated beverages are bad for your health and they should be avoided.

I would like to make a toast now to my readers! Here's to perfect health:Cheers! And cheers to your peers!

k)Sugar

This deadly white poison that has over 100 bad side effects. Here are only 30 reasons why sugar (refined white sugar) is ruining your health or killing you:

1-Sugar can suppress the immune system

2-Sugar upsets the mineral relationships in your body:causes chromium and copper deficiencies and interferes with absorption of calcium and magnesium

3-Sugar can cause a rapid rise of adrenaline,hyperactivity,anxiety, difficulty concentrating and crankiness in children

4-Sugar causes a loss of tissue elasticity and function,the more sugar you eat,the more elasticity and function you lose.

5-Sugar leads to cancer of the breast,ovaries,prostate and rectum

6-Sugar can weaken eyesight.

7-Sugar can increase fasting levels of glucose and can cause reactive hypoglycemia

8-Sugar can cause premature aging. In fact,the single most important factor that accelerates aging is insulin,which is triggered by sugar

9-Sugar can lead to alcoholism

10-Sugar can cause your saliva to become acidic,tooth decay and periodontal disease

11-Sugar contributes to obesity.

12-Sugar can cause many problems with the gastrointestinal tract including:an acidic digestive tract,indigestion, malabsorption in patients with functional bowel disease, increased risk of Crohn's disease, and ulcerative colitis

13-Sugar can cause arthritis.

14-Sugar can cause asthma.

15-Sugar greatly assists the uncontrolled growth of Candida Albicans (yeast infections).

16-Sugar can cause gallstones.

17-Sugar can cause heart disease.

18-Sugar can cause appendicitis.

19-Sugar can cause cancer of the rectum.

20-Sugar can cause multiple sclerosis.

21-Sugar can cause hemorrhoids.

22-Sugar can cause varicose veins.

23-Sugar can contribute to osteoporosis.

24-Sugar can lower the amount of Vitamin E in the blood.

25-Sugar can decrease growth hormone.

26-Sugar can increase cholesterol.

27-Sugar can increase the systolic blood pressure.

28-Sugar can cause drowsiness and decreased activity in children.

29-Sugar can interfere with the absorption of protein.

30-Sugar causes food allergies.

Foods and drinks that contain sugar taste the best but they are the worst. Avoid sugar forever or cut it down to a minimum and if you must use a sweetener use something natural that will not ruin your health like:

organic or cane sugar,honey, stevia, xylitol,etc.

Also,avoid these other poisonous artificial sweeteners: splenda, sweet and low, sucralose,aspartame etc.

No more sugar for you,okay sugar?

l)Microwaved foods

Microwaved foods are making you sick and killing you slowly but surely:

1)The microwave ovens were invented by the Nazis to be used for the invasion of Russia

2)The use of microwave ovens was banned in Russia in 1976 because they were deemed unsafe

3)A woman named Norma Levitt had hip surgery and then she be killed by a simple blood transfusion when a nurse "warmed the blood for the transfusion in a microwave oven"

4)Vegetables and other food lose valuable,cancer-fighting nutrients when cooked in the microwave oven

5)The chemical structure of foods changes when microwaved with unknown consequences
6)Continually eating food processed from a microwave oven causes long term-permanent-brain damage by "shorting out" electrical impulses in the brain (depolarizing or demagnetizing the brain tissue)
7)The human body cannot metabolize (break down) the unknown by-products created in microwaved food.
8)Male and female hormone production is shut down and/or altered by continually eating microwaved foods
9)The effects of microwaved food by-products are residual(long term,permanent) within the human body
10)Minerals,vitamins and nutrients of all microwaved food is reduced or altered so that the human body gets little or no benefit or the human body absorbs altered compounds that cannot be broken down.
11)The minerals in vegetables are altered into cancerous free radicals when cooked in microwave ovens.
12)Microwaved foods cause stomach and intestinal cancerous growths (tumors).This may explain the rapidly increased rate of colon cancer in America.
13)The prolonged eating of microwaved foods causes cancerous cells to increase in human blood
14)Continual ingestion of microwaved foods causes immune system deficiencies through lymph gland and blood serum alterations
15)Eating microwaved food causes loss of memory,concentration,emotional instability and a decrease of intelligence
You know that saying"Kill or be Killed?" You either "kill" your microwave oven or it will kill you. I suggest you microwave your your microwave oven before it microwaves you in the oven!

Trash that deadly appliance ASAP.I did!
m)Meat
There is a saying:"Meat is murder".
Here's my version of that saying:
"Meat is double murder"
First,you are eating a murdered animal and second that dead meat you are eating is murder on your body meaning meat is killing you slowly but surely.
Here are 15 reasons why you should never eat meat:
1-Meat has its own diseases
Even though it is easy to find a disease in an animal and then treat it properly,other chronic diseases are not that easily found. In fact,think about how healthy an animal can be:they spend their entire short life in a tiny cage where cannot even properly stand up,they cannot walk around freely and just like humans,animals need to be loved too but they are not getting any love and they are mistreated and murdered instead,all this in the name of profit.
2-Meat is very hard on the digestive system
Meat can cause a lot of digestive problems. Meat takes a long time to pass through the intestines,where during this time it rots.
Putrefaction produces toxins and amines that accumulate in the liver,kidneys and large intestines and it destroys bacterial cultures and causes degeneration of the lining of the small intestine. After a few years of a regular meat diet,rotting meat will stick to the lining of your intestines,where it often causes various digestive problems such as IBS,stomach cramps, prolapsed colons,hemorrhoids,constipation and many other health problems.
3-Meat contains synthetic hormones

which disturb our hormonal balance. Most farms today inject the animals with different hormones to speed up the animal's growth. The faster the animal grows, the faster the financial return and the bigger it grows the more meat can be obtained for less money.

Most of the hormones are various growth hormones which disrupt our own hormonal balances and this will cause many health problems in your body.

4-Meat contains various drugs

Because animal meat is making certain companies billions of dollars,most or all animals are often injected with many drugs, mostly antibiotics. These drugs do not disappear when the meat is cooked and they end up in your body causing known and unknown diseases. Scientists are still studying the horrible side-effects eating meat inflicts on our bodies.

5-Meat produces toxic compounds when cooked

These are called hetero cyclic amines and they appear in the meat after the meat is cooked,especially at high temperatures.

HCA's(hetero cyclic amines) form when amino acids and creatine react at high cooking temperatures. Scientists have discovered 15 different HCA's resulting from the cooking of muscle meats from beef,pork,chicken and fish.

6-Meat is very high in fat, especially saturated fat

Not all saturated fat is bad but saturated fat from animal meat like meat is bad for your health,especially for your cardiovascular system and your heart. The fat from the meat deposits in the arteries and increases your blood pressure. It can also cause damage your arteries and puts your body at risk for gaining extra unhealthy weight.

7-Meat increases chances of colon cancer

Besides the hetero cyclic amines I talked about earlier,meat does not pass through your intestines fast because meat is high in protein and protein takes a very long time to get fully digested. That means it sits in our intestines the longest and carcinogenic compounds do the most damage to the lining of the intestinal walls which can eventually lead to colon cancer.

8-Meat is very high in calories

Because meat contains so much fat and fat is the most calorie dense nutrient, it is a substance that if it is eaten often or daily,it will definitely lead to weight gain and 300,000 Americans die each year from complications of being overweight.

9-Meat is very high in cholesterol

Most animals produce their own cholesterol and when you eat meat you are increasing your own cholesterol. Your body is capable of regulating its own cholesterol. However,that changes when you ingest the extra cholesterol from animal meats. If you don't wanna be bothered by high cholesterol,then
"don't bother to eat meat"!

10-Meat increases the chances of autoimmune diseases

Due to the fact that some animal proteins are very closely related to ours, the body responds to a lot of these as foreign particles and tries to destroy them. (Not very different from how some organ transplants get rejected.) When the body does this on a regular basis, after some time it begins to turn on itself due to some auto-immune processes that end up resulting in autoimmune diseases.

Got meat? Then don't eat it! Meat? Forget about it!
"One must not deliberately kill any living creature either by committing the act oneself, instructing others to kill or

approving of or participating in acts of killing. To completely abstain from the act of killing directly and indirectly,eat only pure vegetarian food"
Buddhism
n)Foods that your body is allergic to
Most people can eat any foods and be fine but then there is the rest of us who should avoid certain foods. Me for example,I am not allowed to drink cow milk or soy milk and I am not allowed to eat foods that contain:wheat,gluten,oat,barley,etc. To protect your health you should see your natural doctor and you should ask him or her what foods your body is allergic to and avoid them forever.
o)Stress
There is a saying:"Stress is the reason for 85% of diseases out there".That is not true for everybody but is it true for some people. You must live a stress free life if you want a disease free life.
Do not get stressed out for any reason. You must remain calm in all situations if you want all your health!
Mission impossible,huh? Maybe!
What do you call a bee that cannot make up its mind?
A may-bee! (maybe)
Maybe not or maybe nut or maybe nuts...Am I nuts?
p)Amalgam fillings
Amalgam Fillings (Silver or Mercury Fillings)
Did you know that the blood that runs through your tooth will run through your toe within one minute?
The common fillings most people have in their teeth are a mixture of silver,copper,tin and zinc with an equal amount of mercury. Most people's fillings contain more than 60% mercury. Dr. Giamato Plevono has measured

the amount of mercury in ten year old fillings and found it to be 30% mercury. Where does this mercury go? Part of it comes off the surface of a filling in the form of vapor. As we inhale,this vapor enters the lungs and can get into the blood stream. While we eat, it get into our food, then is swallowed,digested and then absorbed into our blood stream. From the blood stream,mercury will get to all organs of our body. Mercury is very toxic. It is a poison in its liquid and vapor forms. Mercury very easily enters our body's cells and can destroy the DNA or nuclear material within those cells.

This can lead to premature aging or reduce resistance. Normal cells live for a short span,then they duplicate themselves. Cells that have been contaminated with mercury die without replacing themselves. After people have removed their mercury fillings,these health problems disappeared:I strongly suggest you see your dentist and have him look for amalgam fillings and he finds any,he should remove them immediately. The more you keep your mercury fillings the more damage they will do to your health.

I suggest you see a natural dentist and have your mercury fillings removed as soon as possible.

WARNING:Before you start your journey to perfect health I need to tell you that you must have these 3 things if you're gonna ever accomplish your mission:

1-You must believe that perfect health is possible for you "Perfect health is perfectly possible"

However,you must be open-minded and believe that anything is possible and nothing is impossible.

2-You must have patience because it's gonna take some time before you enjoy one of the greatest joy there is:

perfect health. It could take months or years before you will achieve your goal of perfect health.

3-You must be financially ready meaning it's not gonna be cheap for most of you to buy natural products or treatments month after month for a while or for the rest of your life.

PS:Remember that success usually doesn't happen over night. Maybe it happens over day! Or over dinner! Or over...That's it. This chapter is over! Wait.not yet. It's not over until the fat lady sings! Or in this case until the fat lady loses weight! The "weight" is over!

How to lose weight without:

Dieting and exercising,Taking any drugs,Having any surgery Here's another lie they've been telling the overweight people for a long ass time:

The only three ways to lose weight are:

1-Diet and exercise 2-Take drugs 3-Have surgery

FACT:

"You can lose weight easily and safely and keep it off forever without dieting,exercising,taking diet pills or having surgery"

Not only do these 3 methods don't work for weight loss but they are dangerous or deadly to your health.

Let's examine them one by one. Ready for the examination of this abomination? Let's get started!

1-Dieting and Exercising

a)Dieting:when you diet you give your body less food and less food means less nutrition. You might lose weight but you will feel hungry and the more you diet the worse you will feel until you quit which is a good thing unfortunately but fortunately you are saving your health or life. When your body gets less nutrition then your body becomes deficient in certain vitamins and minerals and that is definitely gonna make you sick or kill you. You might lose some weight or a lot of weight but after you do you might gain it back or worse:gain more weight back. My advise:Never diet because there isn't one diet in existence today that will help you lose weight safely and keep it off .Fact: Diets don't work

b)Exercising

When you exercise you are burning more calories but if you eat the same amount of food every day,then you are really wasting your time. Besides exercising is not easy and you will feel tired each time you exercise. Let's say that you exercise and you also eat less:it's still not gonna work because your body is starving for good nutrition and when you exercise you are making it worse because the body needs to replace the nutrients you lost when you exercised and there are no nutrients because you are on some low vitamin,low mineral diet. My advise:Don't ever bother to exercise because you are putting your health in danger for nothing and just like dieting,even if you lose weight,you might gain it back or worse:gain more weight back.

2-Taking drugs

All drugs are poison and should never be taken and diet drugs are even more dangerous than regular drugs. Many people have died taking diet drugs or overdosing on them so I strongly suggest you never take any kind of diet drugs to lose weight.

3-Having surgery

That is the worst thing you can do to your body:have surgery on it. Here's another big fat lie:
"Sometimes if you are extremely overweight,you need surgery because it will save your life"

Fact:

You never need surgery to lose weight
Many overweight people died after having surgery to lose weight and many people have suffered irreversible damage from the surgery. If any of the above methods worked,then everybody will be skinny. However,they do work for only 1% of the population or less but keeping the weight off is a different story. You heard the bad new and now it's time to hear the good news!

You have many choices to lose weight easily and safely without:1-Dieting and exercising 2-Taking any diet pills 3-Having any surgery

However,recently I finally found the number one weight loss product in the world,so I'm only gonna talk about that because I will give it to you for free,how about that?

Here are the advantages of this unique breakthrough weight loss product:

1-It is the FASTEST weight loss product in the world
Lose up to 20 pounds in just 10 days!

2-It is the HEALTHIEST weight loss product in the world because:

a)It is organic and 100% natural

b)It is safe for anyone(even if you are taking one or a lot of medications)

c)No hunger and no side-effects

d)Improves your energy level

e)Improves the health of every organ in your body and it also improves your mental health

f)It keeps the body young looking

g)It will make you look and feel better than you ever looked and felt in your life

3-It is the SIMPLEST to use weight loss product in the world because:

a)All you have to do is drink a green drink powder 4 times a day with water or your favorite juice for 10 days from the comfort of your: home,work or anywhere you like

4-It is the LEAST EXPENSIVE weight loss product in the world:around $50 but because:

You are getting it from me,you'll get it for free!

See how much I love you,my lovely readers?

Also,I will give the weight loss product for free to anybody you like and to as many people as you like!

5-After losing all your weight,you have 3 choices:

a)Join the company that has this weight loss product and then you can give it away for free yourself

b)Join the number one health and weight loss company and you can have your own home based business if you like and make as much money as you like!

c)You can also become rich and famous with this company and retire young and rich in about 5 years!

6-This amazing weight loss product has been on the market for 20 years since 1993 and thousands of people have lost weight on it including me! I easily lost 5 lbs in 5 days! And my friend lost 300 lbs in 5 months! Are you next? You could be!

Here is the most health important secret I'll tell you about your health so you can enjoy perfect health forever:

Check your pH at least once a month

As long as your pH is perfect,your health will be perfect too. Enjoy everlasting perfect health!

Tony Davis,P.H.T.
Perfect Health Teacher
Email:SicaBulex@Gmail.com
Http://www.HappyForever.us

www.ingramcontent.com/pod-product-compliance
Lightning Source LLC
Chambersburg PA
CBHW060437290526
45791CB00002B/969

* 9 7 8 1 4 9 5 3 8 7 2 4 1 *